What People Who Take

Vitamin C

Know That You <u>Don't</u>

[handwritten signature/inscription]

Dominick Bosco

Story Hill Books

Story Hill Books
www.DominickBosco.com
db@StoryHillBooks.com

ISBN 13: 978-1505586688

ISBN 10: 1505586682

Printed in the United States of America

"I believe that you can, by taking some simple and inexpensive measures, extend your life and your years of well-being. My most important recommendation is that you take vitamins every day in optimum amounts, to supplement the vitamins you receive in your food."

Linus Pauling

"Vitamins, if properly understood and applied, will help us to reduce human suffering to an extent which the most fantastic mind would fail to imagine."

Albert Szent-Gyorgyi

"Rock & Roll is attitude, burgers, naps, and vitamins."

David Lee Roth

Inside this book:

What People Who Take

Vitamin C

Know That You **Don't**

Vitamin C is the most popular supplement in the world

More people take vitamin C supplements than any other supplement. Researchers called people at random and asked them what supplements they were taking. Out of every 100 people they called, **67** were taking vitamin C.

What do those 67 people know that the other 33 DON'T?

Plenty!

1.

Let's get this over with: Vitamin C CAN help you fight off colds

By far the most talked-about vitamin C subject is its effect on the common cold. Every now and then you still see a magazine or newspaper article in which some misinformed doctor, dietician, or writer claims that there is "simply no evidence" that vitamin C helps prevent or shorten the duration of the common cold.

On the contrary, there has been plenty of evidence for several years.

Back in the 1970s, Linus Pauling claimed that a regular supplement of 1000 mg. (one gram) of vitamin C would significantly reduce the number of colds and days of illness. Responding to those claims, a Canadian epidemiologist, Terence Anderson, M.D., Ph.D., set out to disprove that vitamin C could do any good for cold sufferers. Dr. Anderson put over 800 people on either one gram daily of vitamin C or a placebo. During the first three days of any illness, the volunteers were required to quadruple the dose. Frequency of illness, total days of illness, and number of days of disability (confined to house) were measured and compared.

After fourteen weeks, the vitamin C group had seven percent fewer episodes of illness and twelve percent fewer days of illness. These differences were judged to be not statistically significant, considering the number of people involved in the test. However, one difference was significant: the amount of disability suffered by the vitamin C group was thirty percent less than that of the other group.

A later trial confirmed the results of the first. Using slightly lower doses of vitamin C, people achieved a twenty-five percent reduction in the "days of disability" because of cold symptoms.

So wait, Dr. Anderson's experiments *do* demonstrate that vitamin C undeniably helps people fight off colds.

But they *don't* actually prove that vitamin C prevents colds.

No, but this does:

2.

Yes, vitamin C DOES prevent the common cold. Researchers recently performed what is called a "meta-analysis." They fed the results of over 50 placebo-controlled trials involving over 11,000 people, in which the effects of daily vitamin C supplementation on the incidence, duration, or severity of the common cold were tested. What they found was quite interesting.

It seems that supplementation with vitamin C (250 - 2000 mg. per day) did NOT reduce the frequency of colds in what they called "the general population." But vitamin C supplements DID reduce the number of colds in people with heavy physical stress, such as runners, skiers, or soldiers in subarctic conditions. In these stressed-out people, vitamin C supplements cut frequency of colds in HALF.

Let's talk about this. I no longer run marathons. I don't ski. And I'm not a soldier. But I do exercise. I do shovel snow on occasion. And I do consider myself under stress. These results suggest that there might be some "tipping point" where your stress level is suddenly high enough so you'll benefit from vitamin C supplements. Personally, I don't think nature—my body—works that way. I think stress of any amount raises my vitamin C requirement. I don't really care if I catch one fewer cold a year or not. That's a great benefit if I do, but I think the amount of stress I experience makes me eligible for whatever protection—*from anything*—vitamin C can offer.

These same doctors also found that vitamin C shortened the duration of colds in adults by an average of 8 percent. In children, supplements of 1 to 2 grams per day given when colds began shortened colds by 18 percent. The severity of symptoms was also reduced.

3.

Vitamin C is nothing to sneeze at. Or cough. Another piece of evidence comes from the University of Wisconsin, where researchers selected sixteen healthy students. Half of the students were given 2000 mg. of vitamin C per day, in four equal doses. The other eight received a placebo pill. Three and a half weeks later, all of the students were exposed to people who currently had colds in full bloom. Seven of the eight people in the placebo group came down with colds, and six of the vitamin C group did, too. This difference was really not significant enough to crow about. But there were other differences. The members of the placebo group were sick for an average of twelve days, the vitamin C group only seven days. And the vitamin C group's symptoms were less severe: they had fewer sneezes, fewer coughs, and had to blow their noses less often.

4.

The Australians cooked up a novel way to test vitamin C's effectiveness in battling the common cold. They assembled ninety-five pairs of identical twins, presumably because twins would have identical physiological reactions. One twin from each pair was given one gram of vitamin C per day for 100 days; the other was given a placebo. During the 100 days, the length of time each twin suffered from cold symptoms was measured. Sure enough, the twins who received vitamin C suffered colds of significantly shorter duration than the others.

5.

Vitamin C fights infections by strengthening your immune system. White blood cell levels of vitamin C are known to fall during stress. That stress can include a heart attack, an infection, or simply overwork. Adding extra vitamin C to the diet raises the white blood cell levels back to, and even beyond, normal. Vitamin C has also been shown to boost the activity of the lymphocytes, which are the white blood cells responsible for resisting infecting organisms. It took only 500 mg. of vitamin C per day to stimulate the production of lymphocytes in elderly patients. Vitamin C also reverses the depression of the immune system by steroid drugs.

6.

Vitamin C boosts the body's production of a natural antibacterial, antiviral substance called interferon. Interferon is especially efficient against viruses. If cells attacked by a virus can produce enough interferon, the virus will be prevented from reproducing and the infection will be successfully resisted. Interferon also stimulates at least one other member of the infection-fighting team, the macrophages, which are large cells whose special function is to devour any invading cell, whether it's a virus, bacterium, or cancer cell.

7.

Vitamin C is powerful enough to take on polio. Back as far as the 1930s, before there was a vaccine, vitamin C's effect on the body's resistance to infection was known and studied. In 1935, very high blood levels of vitamin C inactivated poliomyelitis virus and, in animal experiments, provided a small amount of protection against paralysis when the virus was injected into the nervous system.

8.

Vitamin C boosts your antibodies. In healthy young medical students, one gram of vitamin C per day substantially increased blood levels of three of the body's four most important antibodies. Japanese studies have reported vitamin C in high doses is effective against hepatitis, measles, mumps, viral pneumonia, herpes zoster, herpes facialis, stomatitis apthosa, and certain types of meningitis.

9.

Vitamin C boosts the strength of antibiotics. Australian experiments demonstrated that vitamin C not only remarkably enhanced the effect of antibiotics, but that it also enabled certain antibiotics to kill bacteria they previously could not. Many people suffering bacterial infections were helped through this effect, the researchers report.

So, if this book ended here, there's already enough to make me a believer in taking vitamin C supplements.

But there's a LOT more to the vitamin C story....

10.

Most animals make their own vitamin C.
We don't.

So what? So what if every other animal —except monkeys, guinea pigs, fruit-eating bats, and a species of bird—manufactures all the vitamin C they need and humans don't?

Well, for one thing, those animals tend to have higher tissue levels than we do. If you're the suspicious type, as I am, that's a signal that our average levels aren't high enough.

But wait, does evolution make mistakes? Of course it does. It would be great if our bodies made their own vitamin C. It'd be one less thing to worry about. But evolution has left us lots of worries that other animals don't have. We have the ability—and the necessity—to make choices that determine whether we survive, thrive, or die. Cross this street now? Eat this? Jump in that roaring surf? Take vitamin supplements?

11.

When someone uses the words "There's no evidence..." when talking about vitamin C's effects on health, they're misinformed. Vitamin C is one of the most heavily researched substances in the world. There are mountains of studies published in scientific and medical journals. Chances are that if you Google or Bing search for vitamin C and just about any health issue, you will find some research about it. You'll find "evidence." And lots of it. This book is the tip of the tip of the tip of the iceberg of vitamin C "evidence."

Besides, even with "evidence," changes in conventional wisdom and practice can be slow to come, as the next point illustrates:

12.

Vitamin C was not immediately accepted as the cure for scurvy, despite scientific evidence. It took more than 40 years before physician James Lind's research—which, by the way, was the very first controlled study ever conducted—was widely applied to prevent and cure scurvy among British sailors. And it took even longer for the cure to become known in the USA. Over 100 years after Lind's work, people were still needlessly dying of scurvy. As many as 15 percent of deaths during the Civil War were caused by scurvy.

13.

When Vitamin C is low, body and mind come apart at the seams. Vitamin C is way more important than helping us fight off sniffles. At every point in the body where something needs to grow, heal, repair itself, or just maintain its structural integrity—which is just about everywhere— vitamin C must be there in adequate quantities. If it's not, it affects everything. A prolonged vitamin C deficiency results in bleeding, delayed healing, swelling, gum inflammation, loose teeth, swollen joints, anemia, weakness, emaciation, joint and muscle pain, plus neurological symptoms including irritability, hysteria, and depression. Body and mind literally come apart at the seams. This collection of symptoms, in the extreme, is called scurvy.

But what about when the deficiency and the symptoms are not exactly extreme?

14.

Vitamin C is used up when we are stressed. When we are stressed in any way, vitamin C stored in the adrenal glands is discharged into the blood. The excess vitamin C is needed to help us survive the stress. It's no coincidence that one of the symptoms of vitamin C deficiency is a reduced ability to tolerate stress.

15.

Exercised muscles need more vitamin C, because when muscles are worked, they use vitamin C at an increased rate. It's no surprise, then, that muscle weakness and fatigue are symptoms of vitamin C deficiency.

16.

Vitamin C can help infertile women conceive. Doctors in Japan gave 400 mg. of vitamin C to 42 infertile women who were not responding to fertility drugs. Of the women given only vitamin C and no drugs, 14 percent were able to ovulate. Of the women given vitamin C and the drug, 40 percent began to ovulate and slightly more than half of those women became pregnant. It's no coincidence that the ovaries are one of the places in the body where vitamin C is concentrated.

17.

Vitamin C can help infertile men, too. A common cause of male infertility is sperm that sticks together and cannot swim forward to fertilize the egg. A group of thirty-five men with this problem were given 500 mg. of vitamin C every twelve hours. After a month of this treatment, clumping of sperm had been reduced to as low as eleven percent, a percentage high enough for fertility. The men's sperm count, viability, and sperm mobility also improved. In a follow-up, twelve men were given a similar vitamin C dose and, within two months, were able to impregnate their wives.

18.

Can't stand the heat and humidity? Vitamin C can help. Some very curious doctors found that mine workers' vitamin C levels fell during their first few months of working in the hot, humid mines. They wanted to see if supplemental vitamin C would help the workers adjust to the stress. So new mine workers were given either a vitamin C supplement (250 to 500 mg.) or a placebo pill, and observed while they worked in a controlled climate chamber designed to acclimate workers to mine conditions. Vitamin C definitely helped them adjust to the heat, since the internal body temperatures of the supplemented workers were lower than the unsupplemented workers on every day of the test. After four days in the heat, 35 percent of the supplemented workers were fully accustomed to the heat, whereas only five percent of the unsupplemented workers were.

19.

Vitamin C can help with cold sensitivity, too, but only if you take "excessive" amounts. Some researchers had a bug up their butts about vitamin C and stress, so they decided to prove that vitamin C impaired our response to stress. They exposed three groups of guinea pigs to severe cold for about an hour. Remember: guinea pigs, like humans, cannot manufacture their own vitamin C. The guinea pigs that were deficient in vitamin C didn't do so well. They recovered from the cold slowly, and some of them died. The guinea pigs given the guinea pig RDA for vitamin C also didn't fare so well. But the group given "excessive" amounts of vitamin C recovered rapidly, with no lost guinea pigs. So much for proving that vitamin C impairs our stress response! Gimme some of that "impairing."

20.

After surgery, tissue levels of vitamin C drop by as much as forty-two percent. Many doctors and nutritionists recommend supplements of vitamin C for people undergoing surgery or some other process that requires healing. Unfortunately, not all doctors are aware of this advice. One study found blood levels of vitamin C low enough to indicate scurvy in all 1400 surgical patients with infections!

21.

So it makes sense that Vitamin C can help you heal faster. You don't need to have scurvy to benefit from vitamin C. Even if you have "normal" blood levels, vitamin C can help you heal. Ten surgical patients with pressure ulcers were given 500 mg. of vitamin C twice a day, and ten were given a placebo. All twenty had normal and more or less equal blood levels of the vitamin before the supplementation began. Yet the vitamin C-supplemented group healed almost twice as fast as the unsupplemented group.

22.

There are many common situations in which vitamin C can help the body heal faster. A Navy physician found that 600 mg. of vitamin C (plus 600 mg. of bioflavonoid complex) cut the healing time for herpes sores on the lips to less than half when the treatment was begun at the first signs of the infection. Vitamin C supplements (1000 mg.) have been shown to speed the healing of stubborn prickly heat rash, too.

23.

Vitamin C can help relieve back pain. Texas neurosurgeon James Greenwood, MD used doses of vitamin C in excess of 1000 mg. per day on hundreds of people with degeneration of the discs in the lower back. Vitamin C helps the disc connective tissue strengthen and heal, which makes sense since collagen is an important part of connective tissue. Many of his patients were able to completely avoid surgery after vitamin C treatment. He also reported that 1000 mg. of vitamin C per day helps prevent back trouble.

24.

Why your cardiologist is taking vitamin C supplements:

Heart disease patients need more vitamin C. For at least eight weeks after a heart attack, white blood cell levels of vitamin C fall to the levels found in scurvy. This indicates that heart disease patients need more vitamin C after an attack. But what about before the attack? Could vitamin C prevent that attack? No one is claiming that vitamin C can cure heart disease, but there is some research out there that suggests vitamin C could play an important part in a heart disease prevention plan that also includes healthy diet and exercise.

25.

Blocked blood vessels are vitamin C deficient. In the middle of the last century, it was discovered that vitamin C deficiency in guinea pigs produced atherosclerotic lesions that were identical to those of the human disease. But what about humans? The same researchers subsequently measured vitamin C levels in human arteries, and found that arteries with atherosclerotic lesions had much lower levels of vitamin C than arteries free of lesions.

26.

How Vitamin C protects the blood vessels: Atherosclerosis—blocked blood vessels—begins with an attack by free radicals. We know that vitamin C neutralizes those free radicals. It's possible that a localized vitamin C deficiency starts the process by allowing the ground substance of the blood vessels to deteriorate, which then causes the deposit of cholesterol plaques.

27.

Vitamin C lowers cholesterol, triglycerides, and blood pressure. There's a lot of evidence that vitamin C can lower cholesterol and triglycerides. Russian studies in the 1950s found that as little as 500 mg. twice a day, a low-fat diet, abstention from alcohol, and a moderate amount of exercise lowered cholesterol as much as fifty percent. Blood pressure dropped to normal in many patients, and they subsequently could return to a normal life.

Czech doctors gave one gram supplements twice a day to 82 men and women between the ages of 50 and 75. They found that vitamin C did, in fact, lower blood levels of cholesterol, but that the degree of lowering was dependent on how high the levels were in the first place. Persons with low cholesterol levels experienced little or no lowering. In some people with low cholesterol (below 200 mg.), vitamin C appeared to slightly raise their levels. However, in people with cholesterol levels above 230 mg., vitamin C produced a substantial decline in sixty percent of the patients, a decline which persisted for nine months while the experiment was still proceeding and for six weeks after the supplements stopped. The researchers concluded that "chronic, latent vitamin C deficiency" produced the high blood levels of cholesterol.

American researchers succeeded in using vitamin C to lower triglyceride levels from fifty to seventy percent in heart patients.

In elderly men, one gram of vitamin C each day reduced LDL cholesterol levels by as much as fifteen percent. Persons with high levels of triglycerides were given one gram of vitamin C three times a day. After two months, their blood triglycerides were found to be sixty percent lower than when the experiment began.

Blood levels of vitamin C, cholesterol, and triglycerides were measured in 600 fasting blood donors aged twenty-five to fifty-five (half male, half female). For both sexes, the lower their blood levels of vitamin C, the higher were their cholesterol and triglycerides. Normal blood levels of cholesterol and triglycerides were most common in the group with high vitamin C concentration. In fact, a person with high vitamin C levels was two to three times less likely to have high blood fats.

28.

Vitamin C can also raise levels of healthy HDL cholesterol. Doctors at Tufts University found that among 238 elderly people, those who had higher blood levels of vitamin C also had higher levels of HDL cholesterol. In another Tufts study of more than 600 elderly people, similar results were obtained: people who had diets with more than 1000 mg. of vitamin C per day had HDL levels about eight percent higher than those who got fewer than 120 mg. per day, and ten percent higher than those who got fewer than sixty mg. per day.

29.

Vitamin C helps protect against heart attacks by inhibiting blood clots. Several studies have shown that vitamin C inhibits or prolongs the process of platelet aggregation, in which blood platelets group together to form clots. One gram of supplemental vitamin C substantially increased fibrinolytic activity, which prevents clots from forming, even when dietary fat was increased. In a follow-up, one gram doses every eight hours reduced the tendency of the blood platelets to clump together into potentially dangerous clots. This tendency is a major risk factor in cardiovascular disease.

30.

Vitamin C lowers blood pressure. Several studies have consistently found that people with higher blood concentrations of vitamin C have lower blood pressure. In these studies, blood levels of vitamin C are used as a measurement of fruit and vegetable intake, not necessarily vitamin C supplements.

31.

Vitamin C strengthens blood vessels and enhances their flexibility. One of the symptoms of scurvy which James Lind noted was "varicose veins under the tongue." Other doctors have noted the same blood vessel weakness under the tongues of people with low vitamin C levels—but not low enough to cause acute scurvy. The initial lesions in atherosclerosis and cerebrovascular disease are thought to be a similar. Since low vitamin C levels have also been found in persons with capillary fragility, and since one of vitamin C's functions is to maintain the integrity of the blood vessels, it's reasonable to assume that a diet high in vitamin C will afford some increased degree of protection from stroke and other forms of vascular disease by strengthening those blood vessels.

It turns out that vitamin C actually does enhance the flexibility of the blood vessels, allowing them to more readily dilate to allow greater blood flow.

32.

Vitamin C lowers your heart disease risk. The Nurses' Health Study (85,000 women followed for 16 years) found that a daily intake of more than 350 mg. of vitamin C was associated with a 25% or greater reduction in the risk for heart disease. A 2004 investigation of almost 300,000 adults comparing the effect of various antioxidants on heart disease risk found that supplemental vitamin C intake above 700 mg. per day reduced heart disease risk by 25 percent. Other similar studies have had inconsistent results, however. Japanese doctors, for example, found a protective effect in women but not in men. Another test found an effect for dietary vitamin C but not supplements. These inconsistencies could be caused by the limitations of studies that depend on the subjects' ability to recall and report what they've eaten.

To eliminate these inconsistencies, other doctors have actually measured vitamin C levels in the blood of research subjects.

One such study discovered that the higher the blood level of vitamin C, the lower the risk of heart failure. The researchers hastened to add that they were using vitamin C levels as a "marker" of fruit and vegetable intake, not intake of supplements.

33.

Does vitamin C provide "complete protection" against heart disease? Of course it doesn't! What this question really asks is whether it's possible to take enough vitamin C to overcome the effects of a high-fat diet and a low-exercise, high-stress lifestyle. The only reasonable answer to that question is "No." The question we should be asking is whether a high vitamin C diet will help strengthen our defenses against cardiovascular disease. The answer to that, based on the evidence, seems to be "Probably, yes." But don't expect vitamin C to make up for a refusal to acknowledge all the other evidence of what helps people avoid heart and blood vessel disease.

34.

Vitamin C reduces diabetes risk. The EPIC study of over 21,000 men and women discovered that as blood levels of vitamin C go up, the risk of diabetes itself goes down. And two large studies found that high blood levels of vitamin C result in lower levels of hemoglobin A1c, an index of glucose tolerance.

35.

Diabetics need more vitamin C. Diabetics in general, and insulin-dependent diabetics in particular, have been found to have lower-than-normal levels of vitamin C in their blood. This apparent lack of, or increased need for, vitamin C could result in some of the disabling side effects of diabetes. For example, diabetics with high blood levels of cholesterol also tended to have low blood levels of vitamin C. Giving them 500 mg. supplements of vitamin C daily resulted in a "striking decline" in high blood cholesterol and a moderate decline in triglycerides. The doctors who carried out this study concluded that vitamin C supplements corrected the local tissue's vitamin deficiency, and improved the liver's ability to metabolize cholesterol into harmless by-products.

36.

Vitamin C lowers risk of diabetes complications. Indian doctors found that supplements of 1000 mg. vitamin C per day given to diabetics reduced blood levels of fasting blood sugar, insulin, LDL cholesterol, and HbA1c. They concluded: "Our results indicate that daily consumption of 1000 mg. supplementary vitamin C may be beneficial in decreasing blood glucose and lipids in patients with type 2 diabetes and thus reducing the risk of complications."

37.

Bruise less with Vitamin C. Diabetics frequently suffer the effects of increased capillary fragility: easy bruising and bleeding. When the diabetic's diet contains "normal" amounts of vitamin C, capillary strength is not increased. However, supplements of one gram of vitamin C restore capillary strength to normal.

38.

Lower your risk of cataracts with Vitamin C. Another researcher has suggested that supplements of vitamin C could help prevent cataracts in diabetics. Animal experiments (guinea pigs) have demonstrated that cataracts develop predominantly in diabetic animals fed a vitamin C-deficient diet.

39.

Will Vitamin C Prevent Cancer?

In the 1970s and 80s, Linus Pauling, Scottish surgeon Ewan Cameron, and other researchers studied vitamin C's effectiveness as a treatment for cancer. Using high doses of vitamin C administered intravenously, they succeeded in improving the quality of life and extending the survival times of terminal cancer patients, some of whom survived for many years.

In an attempt to disprove Pauling and Cameron's claims that vitamin C had a role to play in cancer treatment, a study was performed at the Mayo Clinic. However, the researchers did not follow the same procedures as Pauling and Cameron. Patients were given vitamin C orally instead of intravenously, and only for a limited period of time. The Mayo Clinic researchers declared that vitamin C had no role in cancer treatment, which is precisely what they set out to do. At the time, Pauling noted that none of the Mayo Clinic cancer patients died while receiving vitamin C.

Linus Pauling, the only person to ever win two unshared Nobel Prizes, each in a different category, had a hard time getting the National Cancer Institute to grant funds to carry on more research on vitamin C and cancer. Such was, and is, the power of not only vested interests but also stubborn resistance to new and different ideas. Still, research has been done and is still being done, and it is showing some promise.

Recent research at the University of Kansas has found that when administered intravenously along with conventional chemotherapy, vitamin C reduces the toxic effects of the drugs and does help kill the cancer cells. Other research has shown that vitamin C selectively kills certain cancer cells while not harming regular cells.

40.

So...will vitamin C strengthen your resistance to cancer? The challenge in proving that vitamin C helps prevent cancer is that no actual tests are ever likely to be done in which people are given a high dose or a placebo for years and years and observed to see who gets cancer and who doesn't. The studies that are done usually involve amounts of vitamin C more in line with what a conventionally "healthy" diet might provide, in the 100 - 200 mg. range. And even then, the actual vitamin C in the diet is only estimated from the person's self-reporting of how much fresh fruit and vegetables they eat each day—or, even less reliably, their recollection of how much they ate in the past.

Still, within those limitations, the evidence tends to support the idea that the more vitamin C in your diet, the lower your risk of cancer.

41.

Vitamin C appears to help prevent stomach cancer and gastric cancer. Numerous researchers report that people with gastric cancer tend to have diets lower in vitamin C, and lower in foods containing vitamin C such as fresh fruits and vegetables. Many researchers attribute the decline in gastric cancer in the United States to the overall increased intake of vitamin C. This makes sense because vitamin C is known to inhibit the formation of carcinogenic compounds that enter the stomach through food and certain drugs. Vitamin C supplementation has also been found to reduce the risk of gastric cancer caused by infection with the carcinogenic H. pylori bacterium.

42.

Vitamin C might help prevent colon cancer. Several researchers have reported that vitamin C can help keep rectal polyps from developing into malignant tumors. People with familial polyposis are generally at high risk for development of malignant cancer of the rectum. Surgical removal of the polyps usually gives only temporary relief, since the polyps recur soon thereafter. Treatment with vitamin C, however (one gram, three times a day, in a time-release capsule), resulted in regression of the polyps in five out of eight people. The doctors believe that vitamin C neutralizes carcinogenic chemicals in the colon, which are formed by a bacteria working on the contents of the intestine. Increasing vitamin C intake, eating more bran, and lowering fat in the diet also resulted in a decrease in the amount of potentially carcinogenic material in the colon among people not necessarily suffering from polyposis.

So if you're taking vitamin C supplements and someone remarks that all you're doing is making expensive, vitamin-rich poop, tell them, "You bet. That's the idea!"

More recently, researchers pooled data from over a dozen studies, involving over 676,000 people, and found that higher total intake of vitamin C—in other words, from food AND supplements—did reduce colon cancer risk. The reduction in risk was modest but statistically significant.

43.

Vitamin C might reduce breast cancer risk. A study of over 82,000 female nurses found that premenopausal women with a family history of breast cancer whose diet contained an average of 205 mg/day of vitamin had a 65 percent lower risk of breast cancer than those whose diets contained only 70 mg. Other studies have had mixed results. Some have shown a mild protective effect of higher vitamin C levels, some have not. Those studies involved fewer women than the Nurses Health Study.

44.

Vitamin C might help protect women against cervical cancer. Doctors surveyed the dietary levels of vitamin C in the diets of eighty women who had Pap smears. The thirty-four women who had normal results on the Pap smears were found to have relatively high intakes of vitamin C. But the forty-six women who had abnormal Pap smears—indicating troubles ranging from mild inflammation to actual cancer—were found to have significantly less vitamin C in their diets. The exact role vitamin C plays in protecting the cervix is not known.

Other studies have shown that cervical cancer patients have lower-than-normal blood and tissue levels of vitamin C. It might be that the cervical dysplasia—the growth of abnormal cells in the cervix—itself increases the body's need for the vitamin.

45.

Vitamin C reduces lymphoma risk. The Iowa Women's Health Study collected data on diet and supplement use in 35,159 women (aged 55-69 years) and discovered that higher dietary intake of vitamin C and other antioxidants reduced the risk of developing Non-Hodgkins lymphoma after 19 years of follow-up. The Women's Health Initiative also found that higher total vitamin C intake from diet and supplements reduced the risk of diffuse B-cell lymphoma, a subtype of Non-Hodgkins Lymphoma.

46.

Vitamin C makes you friendlier!

A British study of the effects of low doses of vitamin supplements (100 mg. of vitamin C) found a relationship between high concentrations of vitamin C and increased friendliness and warmth, better concentration, and improved sleep patterns.

47.

Vitamin C makes you more alert. A Czech study found that vitamin C supplements (one gram per day) improved the "vigilance" of a group of coal miners, resulting in fewer accidents and injuries on the job. American doctors found that children from matched pairs of twins given from 500 to 1000 mg. of vitamin C a day for five months not only demonstrated greater resistance to colds, but also increased growth and mental alertness.

48.

Vitamin C fights fatigue. Men and women who were surveyed about their intake of vitamins and their health revealed that those who consumed more than 400 mg. of vitamin C each day had about half as much fatigue as the people who got less than 100 mg. per day in their diet.

49.

Vitamin C supplements could help prevent cataracts. When vitamin C levels in the eye are low, cataracts are more severe. And research has shown a decreased risk of cataracts as vitamin C levels in the diet and tissues increase. In women, at least, tests show taking vitamin C supplements of at least 300 mg. per day for 10 years or more can cut cataract risk by more than half.

50.

Vitamin C, in combination with other antioxidants, can slow the progression of macular degeneration. Advanced macular degeneration was slowed by 25 percent and visual acuity loss by 19 percent when taking 500 mg. per day of vitamin C with vitamin E and zinc.

51.

Vitamin C also reduces pressure in the eye that leads to glaucoma. A large dose is capable of reducing the pressure inside the eyeball within a matter of hours, whereas a dose as small as 500 mg. twice a day succeeded in lowering pressure after two weeks.

52.

Vitamin C helps prevent osteoarthritis arthritis and knee pain. The Framingham osteoarthritis study found that people whose diets contained high amounts of vitamin C had three-fold lower risk of osteoarthritis progression. They also had much lower risk of knee pain.

53.

Vitamin C might also help with rheumatoid arthritis. Researchers found a significant difference in how much vitamin C people with arthritis consumed compared to those who did not develop arthritis. People whose diets had the lowest amounts of vitamin C were three times more likely to develop rheumatoid arthritis than people who consumed the highest amounts of vitamin C.

54.

It's no big surprise that vitamin C can help with arthritis. Because it's an antioxidant, it can neutralize free radicals and other chemicals in the body that trigger inflammation. Vitamin C is also crucial in synthesis of joint tissue and bone.

Also, low vitamin C levels in the tissues increase the chances for and intensity of the allergic response, and that increased concentration of vitamin C could act as an anti-inflammatory agent." Another study found that a combination of vitamin C, bioflavonoids, and enzymes was more effective in reducing inflammation than seven non-steroid anti-inflammatory drugs. And Canadian doctors found that high concentrations of vitamin C (in test tube cultures) were more effective than aspirin in reducing the growth of arthritic cells. Vitamin C completely destroyed the arthritic cells, whereas aspirin merely inhibited their growth."

55.

Vitamin C detoxifies alcohol. Vitamin C helps protect the body from the effects of several common poisons and pollutants. Vitamin C (in doses equivalent to several grams for a human) completely protected animals from the effects of lethal doses of alcohol. All of the vitamin C-treated animals survived the lethal dose, but only thirty percent of the other animals did. The researchers concluded that vitamin C accelerated the clearance of alcohol from the bloodstream.

Further animal experiments have confirmed that vitamin C helps protect the body against the toxic effects of alcohol. Blood levels of alcohol decline faster when animals are given a diet with higher-than-normal amounts of vitamin C. As might be expected, the animals that did not receive vitamin C showed more physical evidence of alcohol toxicity, in the form of fatty changes in the liver.

The authors of the study concluded that a diet which is nutritionally adequate may no longer be so in the presence of high ethanol intake, and that supplemental vitamin C ingestion may afford protection against ethanol toxicity.

Of course, this is significant to anyone who consumes alcoholic beverages. But its significance does not stop there. This study, which was performed at a veterans hospital and the University of Oklahoma College of Medicine, is but one more piece of evidence that vitamin C helps the body deal with toxic substances and that what we normally think of as an "adequate" amount of the vitamin is really not adequate at all. We need more vitamin C to really help protect ourselves from all the toxic influences in today's environment.

56.

Vitamin C helps protects us from cadmium. Strangely enough, we can't live without cadmium. It's an essential nutrient—but in ultra-trace amounts. Unfortunately, it's also an industrial pollutant, so there's way too much of it in our air, water, food, and just about everything else. Cadmium is not only impossible to avoid, but insidious in its effects: kidney damage with resultant high blood pressure, anemia, and gastrointestinal dysfunction resulting in malabsorption of nutrients. Several studies have shown that low levels of vitamin C in the diet and body tissues correspond to higher susceptibility to cadmium toxicity. In quail fed toxic amounts of cadmium, vitamin C supplementation completely prevented the toxic effects of the poison.

In experiments with rats, feeding them vitamin C and iron supplements not only prevented the toxic effects of cadmium, but also reversed toxicity in animals already experiencing them.

57.

Vitamin C also helps protect the body against lead poisoning. Vitamin C supplements (with zinc) dropped the blood levels of lead in workers at a storage battery factory—while the men were still on the job and exposed to lead every day.

58.

Vitamin C protects us against some of the toxic effects of steroid drugs, which include depressed immunity to infections, and slow wound healing. Paracetamol (commonly known as acetaminophen) can cause liver dysfunction and damage. However, 500 mg. of vitamin C, three times a day, protected even undernourished male volunteers given high doses of paracetamol from this effect. Vitamin C protected mice from lethal doses of the drug in another experiment by the same researchers.Since many people take this drug for chronic conditions, it would seem to be a good idea if vitamin C were included in the tablet formulation. Dream on.

59.

Vitamin C and other common pollutants. Vitamin C helps detoxify vanadium (an industrial pollutant), PCB's (polychlorinated biphenyl),and organophosphate insecticides (parathion and malathion).

60.

Vitamin C also helps protect the lungs against air pollution. People were given either 2000 mg. of vitamin C per day or a placebo, then exposed to either clean air or air tinged with nitrogen dioxide, a common air pollutant that causes the body's airways to become more sensitive and irritable. The researchers found that vitamin C prevented the usual irritable response to nitrogen dioxide.

61.

Asthmatics breathe easier with vitamin C. Vitamin C can reduce the choking off of airways induced in asthmatics by exercise. The improvement in breathing can be as high as 50 percent.

62.

Vitamin C makes your hot dog safe to eat.

Nitrosamines are cancer-causing substances formed from nitrates and nitrites in foods. These chemicals are added as preservatives in many processed foods, especially smoked meats. Vitamin C prevents the formation of nitrosamines when it is present in the stomach at the same time as the nitrites or nitrates. One gram per day of vitamin C significantly reduced the levels of cancer-causing nitrosamines in the gastric juice of seven out of eight subjects. Several studies have shown that vitamin C also protects against another toxic effect of nitrates in processed food, a blood disorder called methemoglobinemia.

63.

Vitamin C magically makes chlorinated water taste like it comes from a clear mountain spring! One handy use of vitamin C is to dechlorinate water. A pinch of powdered vitamin

C added to a gallon of water will instantaneously neutralize the chlorine. The taste and odor of the chlorine will also disappear.

64.

Vitamin C enhances absorption of other vital nutrients.
Vitamin C taken with iron (contained in food or in a supplement) increases the absorption of the mineral by as much as 1000 percent, depending on the amount of vitamin C taken and the content of the food. The researchers who carried out this experiment concluded that a 300 mg. supplement of vitamin C taken only at breakfast would increase iron absorption over the day by a factor of two, but that dividing the dose over the day would increase absorption by a factor of three. Vitamin C also enhances absorption of calcium and certain essential amino acids.

65.

Vitamin C blocks the destruction of the B-vitamin thiamin by tannin, if present at the beginning of the reaction. And it reverses the reaction if added to the contents of the gut within a half hour.

66.

Vitamin C converts toxic chromium to safe chromium.
Chromium in its trivalent molecular form is an essential nutrient. But in its hexavalent form, it's toxic. Vitamin C converts hexavalent chromium to trivalent chromium.

67.

How Much Vitamin C Should You Take?

The RDA of vitamin C is way low. The RDA for vitamin C ranges from 40 mg. for infants to 90 mg. for adult males, 80 - 85 mg. for pregnant women, and 120 mg. for lactating women. These amounts seem puny compared to the doses of the vitamin used in experiments described here. Is it possible that so small an amount can fulfill the requirement for all the functions vitamin C apparently has? And does it even make sense that the requirement for a man is higher than that for a pregnant woman?

68.

The RDA for vitamin C is only the amount that will prevent the development of extreme scurvy in normal people. By "scurvy," the scientists who set the standard mean the extreme form, where the body is dramatically and visibly coming apart at the seams. But many doctors and researchers feel that a less extreme, subclinical chronic scurvy can occur with a more insidious development of symptoms, or that localized scurvy can occur in certain areas or tissues of the body, resulting in a whole range of possible disorders.

The symptoms of subclinical scurvy won't be the same in everyone. Some people will suffer reduced immunity. Some will heal slowly from injuries or surgery. Some will be infertile... etc. There is enough evidence to convince several scientists and doctors that "chronic, latent scurvy is prevalent" in modern society. This means that many people are not getting enough vitamin C to help build their resistance to diseases as minor as bleeding gums and easy bruising, or as devastating as cancer and heart disease.

69.

Many factors can contribute to a vitamin C deficiency or an increased need for the vitamin. For example, vitamin C deficiencies have been found in people who don't like acidic foods. Smokers, as a rule, have lower tissue levels of vitamin C than nonsmokers. Smoking is known to directly deplete vitamin C levels (the RDA for smokers is a little higher). This depletion could be one factor in smokers' higher death rate from cancer and heart disease.

70.

Hospital patients have low blood levels of vitamin C, resulting from either the stress of treatment or disease or the inadequacy of hospital nutrition. A check of vitamin C content in a home for the elderly found there wasn't enough to meet even the low RDA.

71.

Babies in America have scurvy. Infants fed on cow's milk, without supplementation with vitamin C or fresh orange juice, make up the largest single group of humans with clinically recognized scurvy in the United States and Canada. Breastfed infants, on the other hand, have an extremely low rate of scurvy.

72.

Vitamin C levels are lower than normal in people with liver disease, a deficiency which can result in an increase in the toxicity of drugs used to treat the disease. Hyperthyroid patients also tend to have lower than normal tissue levels of vitamin C.

Several drugs can cause a vitamin C deficiency. Among them are: adrenal corticosteroids (which can actually induce scurvy symptoms); estrogen-containing drugs such as oral contraceptives and menopausal drugs; barbiturates; and tetracycline. Aspirin can increase urinary excretion of vitamin C by a factor of three.

73.

Any condition which results in an increase in blood levels of copper can also increase the need for vitamin C. Many people are not aware that considerable copper can enter the body through water which is piped through copper plumbing. Apparently, vitamin C is involved in the detoxification of excess levels of copper.

74.

What do the experts say? All of these facts don't really answer the question of how much vitamin C we need in our diet or through supplementation. And it doesn't make answering it any easier—although it may reduce your anxiety—to realize that the experts can't agree, either. Not even the scientists who agree that we need more than the RDA of vitamin C, nor those who agree that we need more than our food can practically provide, agree on just how much we should take.

75.

Animals who synthesize their own vitamin C will make more of the vitamin when they are stressed. For example, when a rat is stressed, its vitamin C production triples. A human would have to take several grams to equal such a boost in vitamin C available to the tissues.

76.

Dr. Roger J. Williams answered the question by saying that it depends on how much we consider we "need" and how much we consider "a luxury." Dr. Williams, one of the pioneers of nutritional research, said one level of intake will prevent acute scurvy, and that condition might be considered "health" by some people. But many people aren't satisfied with that, and want "better" health, or "optimal" health. One of the things these people who want optimal health will do is get more vitamin C.

But, Williams noted, because of wide variations in requirements among individuals, what helps create optimum health for one person might not be enough for another.

77.

Wait—there are experts who say we can get all our vitamins from food! This is the fantasy that will not die! We cannot get all our necessary nutrients from food alone. Period. Our food supply and the information we receive about it is hopelessly corrupted by corporate influence. The food industry and the pharmaceutical industry can buy all the science, all the academics, and all the government agencies it needs to not only influence regulations on what constitutes a "nutritional requirement" but also how nutrition is taught to professionals in universities as well as to children in schools.

The food industry has a huge stake in keeping officially recognized nutritional requirements as low as possible. And they do. Processed food, genetically modified food, badly stored food, food created in a factory with as few nutrients as possible for longer shelf life... all these things make a mockery of any claim to "science."

The fact that the agriculture-food industry lobby can prevent labeling of genetically modified foods—something an overwhelming majority of Americans want—is proof that our system of government regulation and official advice about nutrition is hopelessly corrupted and unreliable.

78.

But would nature leave us in such a situation? Of course it would! Is it "natural" to need 500 or 1000 or 5000 mg. of vitamin C in order to be healthy? Who defines "natural" anyway? The RDA is not based on natural facts or observations, but on arbitrary decisions by a committee, influenced by economic and political factors, not just pure science.

Nature's requirements are not based on what's fair, or politically or economically profitable. Primitive people, who might be considered closer to nature, ate a diet that was much higher in vitamin C than the modern diet. They ate their fruits and vegetables fresh and raw. When they ate meat, they ate the organs that were highest in vitamin C first and left the muscle meats for last. Many nutritional scientists and archaeologists believe that the reason people have a preference for sweet-tasting food is that in nature sweet-tasting foods (fruits, particularly) are rich in vitamin C.

And yet we are bombarded by more stresses and trauma than our ancestors. Different kinds of stresses. Our ancestors had to worry about infections, but not about chemical pollutants. Plus, our ancestors roaming around in a state of paleo-purity, rarely lived past 40.

79.

Modern life isn't "natural." Asking this question, "Would Nature leave us in the lurch like this, unable to manufacture something we need to live a healthy life?" doesn't do us any good. It assumes Nature somehow revolves around us and everything that happens in Nature is for our benefit. Not true.

Nature didn't provide us with a lot of things we have come to depend on in this life. And, besides, there are plenty of things out there that are decidedly unnatural, like PCBs and other pollutants. Nature didn't intend for us to live in a world where thousands of toxic chemicals pollute our air, water, and food.

80.

Here is just a single example of such a toxin. Perfluorooctanoic acid (PFOA) is an industrial, man-made chemical that is a confirmed cancer-causing toxin. It's toxic to the liver, the immune system, and the endocrine system. It's linked to infertility, hyperactivity, late onset of puberty, and several cancers. Research has shown PFOA has a definite roll in causing kidney cancer, testicular cancer, ulcerative colitis, thyroid disease, high cholesterol, and high blood pressure during pregnancy. And unless you're one of the lucky 2%, you have it in your body. I'll say that again: 98% of the US population has PFOA in their bodies. It's in carpets, microwave popcorn bags, cleaning fluids, nonstick cookware, water-repellant fabrics, food, wax paper, clothing, upholstery, floor wax, sealants for stone, wood, and tile, dental floss, candy wrappers....

And in case you're thinking you never use any of these, you still have to breathe and drink. It's in the air and water, too. And in case you're thinking of moving to a desert island, you still won't escape PFOA. It's on every continent and in ocean water, even the middle of the Pacific.

PFOA is just one of thousands of industrial chemicals in our air, water, food, and clothing. Vitamin C probably doesn't protect us against all of them, or even very many of them. But it DOES help protect us against SOME of them. And though I didn't expect that PFOA was one of them, it turns out that it just might be. I searched for "PFOA and vitamin C" and discovered that in one study, a combination of vitamin C, glucan, and resveratrol offered significant immune system protection against PFOA in laboratory tests with mice.

81.

OK, here's another: lead in cigarette smoke. Researchers were surprised to find that 1000 mg. supplements of vitamin C reduced blood lead levels from cigarette smoke by over 80 percent—but 200 mg. supplements or placebo had no effect. So much for the canard "any dose over 200 mg. does no good whatsoever!" What's even more interesting about this discovery is that blood levels of vitamin C in both supplemented groups were about the same. The extra 800 mg. per day did not raise blood levels of the vitamin, despite the fact that it was reducing lead levels. Vitamin C works in mysterious ways.

82.

Saturate your body with vitamin C? Many researchers cite the amount of vitamin C necessary to maintain tissue saturation as the optimally required dose. Under normal, unstressed circumstances, 120 mg. usually suffices. (If you're living in a perfectly constructed bubble.) But this requirement rises considerably during any kind of stress. (If you're living in the real world.) Furthermore, this might not take into account that local tissue deficiencies of vitamin C can require many times more vitamin C than it takes to saturate other parts of the body. (See No.81 above.)

Remember, in many of the experimental therapeutic uses of vitamin C, the affected tissues were often deficient in vitamin C even when blood and other tissue levels were normal. In a test of the effect of vitamin C on elderly hospital patients, one gram was given daily to a group which was found to have blood plasma and leukocyte levels of vitamin C that "overlapped" with those seen in scurvy. The daily dose of vitamin C did improve their health and well-being, but their leukocyte levels of the vitamin still did not rise all the way to normal.

83.

More evidence that the RDA for vitamin C is not high enough: Doctors investigating vitamin C and gum health found dietary levels of vitamin C that were equal to or lower than the RDA resulted in gum bleeding. But at 600 mg. per day of vitamin C, gum bleeding was reduced significantly. (BTW: If your gums are in bad shape, it may not even take that much vitamin C supplementation to help. In persons with particularly low intake of vitamin C, between twenty and forty mg. per day, supplementation with as little as seventy mg. per day can be sufficient to begin the healing process in diseased gums.)

The more research reports you read, the more it seems that the RDAs are ridiculously low.

84.

But really, how much should you take? Linus Pauling recommended taking at least 2 grams per day. He also recommended increasing the dose until "looseness of the bowels" occurred and then backing off until it stopped. That, he believed, was the best way to determine your optimal dose.

85.

Linus Pauling wasn't the only Nobel winner to take vitamin C supplements. Dr. Albert Szent-Gyorgyi, 1937 Nobel laureate in Medicine, who won for his scientific work on vitamin C, confided to Pauling that he took 1000 mg. per day.

86.

Pauling based his recommendations on several factors. He analyzed the amount of vitamin C synthesized by mammals that could make their own, and found that a 100-pound goat synthesized about 9 grams per day. He also measured the amount of vitamin C primates actually ate—since, like humans, these evolutionary relatives also do not make their own. He found that 400 pound gorillas consume between 3 and 6 grams per day.

87.

Pauling also calculated the amount of vitamin C supplied by a day's worth of raw fruit and vegetables— enough to add up to 2500 calories. Presumably, this would be the amount you would get if you ate a completely natural diet. He came up with over 2 grams—38 times the RDA.

88.

My personal daily supplement is 2 - 3 grams, but that's not arrived at by any specific process. On occasion, in times of increased stress or when fighting off a cold, I will take additional doses of 500 - 1000 mg.

   Shhh... don't tell anyone... but once every 4 weeks, I set up all my vitamin supplements in pill minder boxes. Every now and then I get to the end of my 4 weeks and feel too lazy to set them all up again. On those rare days, I still always take my usual dose of vitamin C.

89.

Precise requirement? Is there an app for that? I don't think it will ever be possible to come up with a way to determine your precise need for vitamin C or any other nutrient. Even if you had an app on your phone that could analyze every cell in your body and tell you how much you needed, it wouldn't account for the bad news you might get at work...or the guy who sneezes in your face on the subway... or the flat tire you have to change in the rain coming home.

90.

Vitamin C is not toxic!

I'm weary of reading click bait about "risky" vitamin C. It's always a sign the writer hasn't done enough homework. Vitamin C is not toxic. I could find no evidence of people admitted to emergency rooms because of vitamin C toxicity. There are, however, tens of thousands of ER visits and hospital admissions yearly for aspirin, acetaminophen, ibuprofen, and other common over-the-counter drugs. For acetaminophen alone, the number of ER visits per year exceeds 50,000.

91.

It's so widely known that acetaminophen can kill you that it is a favorite drug-of-choice for suicide attempts. It is the most common cause of acute liver failure. Only about 2/3 of those 50,000 cases of poisoning are intentional. The rest are unintentional: parents giving their children a little too much of the medicine the doctor told them to give them, adults taking an extra dose or two because their doctors and the TV commercials have given them the impression that it's safer than aspirin. The difference between a "recommended dose" of acetaminophen and a liver-damaging toxic dose can be as little as a single extra dose.

92.

Yet there are NO reports of vitamin C overdose, emergency room visits, or hospital admissions. Zero. For the most popular supplement on the planet. Millions of people taking tons of the stuff and no reports of toxicity. Hmmm... I guess it's pretty safe.

All the handwringing articles about vitamin C's "toxicity" are based on speculation and sketchy lab tests. They're not based on any actual clinical experience. Nobody goes to the hospital with "vitamin C overdose."

So why do these articles keep appearing with the fear-mongering headlines? Because that's the way the media works. They want to attract interest, and the time-tested way to do that is to raise an alarm and warn people about some danger—real or imagined.

Media reports of vitamin C's toxicity and speculation of its toxicity by some doctors are ungrounded in fact. Reports of its intravenous use in humans at doses ranging from a few grams to over 200 grams all agree that no serious side effects are produced. And even at those high doses, the supposed diuretic effects of vitamin C were not observed by Dr. Pauling, Dr. Cameron or their colleagues.

93.

What about "the rebound effect?" One effect of high doses of vitamin C that is still controversial is the so-called "rebound" effect, in which a person taking high doses will become deficient in the vitamin when the dosage is suddenly reduced. Some studies have shown that the body "adjusts" to very high intake of vitamin C by becoming less efficient in absorbing it and more efficient in excreting it. If this were so, suddenly dropping from a high dose to a low dose could rapidly deplete body stores. Although some tests have shown that there is no "rebound" effect and that body stores remain high long after long-term high doses (two grams per day), higher doses might require gradual "weaning" to a lower daily dose.

94.

What actually happens when you take "too much" vitamin C? By now, decades after Linus Pauling recommended high doses of vitamin C, just about everyone should know that high doses can cause flatulence, bloating, diarrhea, and gas. These side effects are not normally harmful. They are just a sign that your body doesn't need quite as much vitamin C as you're giving it at that time. In fact, as noted above, Pauling suggested this was the best way to discover your optimum dose.

To avoid this effect and still take high doses, you might want to try distributing the dose over several smaller doses throughout the day. Calcium ascorbate and sodium ascorbate might not produce this effect.

95.

Does vitamin C increase your chances of developing kidney stones? This is the "toxic effect" most commonly used to try to scare people away from vitamin C supplements—unsuccessfully, since it is far and away the most commonly taken supplement, with millions of people taking billions of milligrams every day. That fact alone is usually enough to give the lie to any claims that vitamin C might actually increase kidney stone risk. With so many people taking large amounts, if there were any truth to the claim, we would see an epidemic of kidney stones among vitamin C users. No such epidemic—or even sporadic outbreaks—ever materialized. And now we know why....

The attack on vitamin C was based on supposed scientific evidence that vitamin C raises urinary oxalate levels. Oxalate levels are often used as a barometer of one's risk for developing kidney stones. But now we have a study which not only reveals that vitamin C does NOT raise urinary oxalate levels, but also explains why earlier evidence said it did.

A number of people were given eight grams of vitamin C per day. When their blood and urine levels of oxalate were measured before, during, and after the vitamin C supplementation period, the levels did not rise significantly above pre-supplementation levels.

Why did the earlier evidence show an increase in oxalate with vitamin C? Old-fashioned lab techniques required heating the sample. New, high-tech methods do not require heating the specimen. Comparing the two methods revealed that it's heating the sample that artificially raises oxalate levels, not vitamin C. Another test confirmed these results. Healthy male volunteers were given ten grams of vitamin C per day in two gram doses. Their oxalate levels did rise slightly, but as the doctors who carried out the test said: "The increase ... was very low, and is thus similar to the change in urinary content of oxalate which results from consuming normal diets."

Another factor in stone formation is inflammation caused by high uric acid levels. But vitamin C actually *reduces* uric acid levels and has actually been shown to prevent gout, which is also caused by high uric acid levels.

96.

Where do you get your vitamin C?

The richest natural sources of vitamin C are raw fruits and vegetables. Several vegetables, such as red and yellow peppers, actually have more vitamin C than oranges and other citrus. But these foods are not always eaten raw. (Once they're cooked, say bye bye to the vitamin C.) And because they don't store as well as citrus, they were not used on ships to prevent scurvy—so they didn't get the reputation for being good sources of vitamin C.

Vitamin C levels in fresh foods vary according to how they're grown, stored, and prepared. The amount of sunlight determines vitamin C content, more sunlight producing more of the vitamin. Vitamin C is vulnerable to oxidation, so storage can expose it to considerable losses. Since the vitamin is water-soluble, steaming for prolonged periods, washing, soaking, and canning result in severe losses. Storage of citrus juice at warm temperatures results in almost total loss of vitamin C content. Frozen orange juice concentrate can have a higher vitamin C content than fresh squeezed—if the oranges are juiced and frozen immediately after picking.

Vitamin C is available in supplemental form in a wide range of doses, from a few milligrams to more than one gram (1000 mg.).

97.

What are we talking about when we're talking about vitamin C? I've seen claims that synthetic vitamin C is not really vitamin C at all, and that the entire constellation of cofactors and bioflavonoids present in natural sources must be present for "vitamin activity" to take place. Well, it depends who is doing the talking. Linus Pauling and most other scientists who performed research on vitamin C definitely were referring to synthetic vitamin C. There is no practical way to get several grams of vitamin C into your diet without using synthetic vitamin C. To get two grams naturally, you would need to eat around 30 fresh oranges... or 10 cups of raw chili peppers... or 12 cups of raw red peppers...or 25 cups of fresh papaya...or from 50 grams to 200 grams of acerola berries, depending on the freshness of the acerola.

98.

What about all those natural cofactors that accompany the vitamin in food? Of course there is a value in also getting the cofactors and bioflavonoids that accompany vitamin C in food. Real food has real nutritional value, and our science is not capable of artificially reproducing and supplying all of the required elements in food.

But vitamin C tablets advertised as "natural" or "rose hips" or "acerola" should be carefully examined before purchase. To achieve high doses, these forms of vitamin C can be composed of synthetic vitamin C with the addition of smaller quantities of acerola berry or rose hips. You're not getting a megadose constructed entirely of "natural" vitamin C.

99.

There's nothing wrong with "synthetic" vitamin C. It's produced by the fermentation of glucose, basically the same way it's produced in nature. However, "natural" vitamin C tablets are often sold for many times the price of the same strength tablet labeled plainly "ascorbic acid."

100.

Vitamin C is also available as sodium ascorbate and calcium ascorbate. Both are sometimes used interchangeably with ascorbic acid in many experiments and therapeutic trials. Persons wishing to keep the sodium in their diet as low as possible would be wise to avoid sodium ascorbate, however. Vitamin C is also available in pure powdered form, which is by far the least expensive way to obtain the vitamin.

And finally...

101.

Take vitamin C and live longer

Back in the middle of the last century—wow, that sounds so forever ago—there were some studies that attempted to parse out if taking vitamin supplements gave you a longer life. Overall, the answer was Yes. I've always thought these studies were kind of naive and quaint—relics of a bygone day.

So I was surprised to find that serious researchers are still doing this kind of research—well into the 21st century! In one study of over 50,000 people aged 50 - 76, taking vitamin C supplements seemed to decrease risk of mortality for five years of follow-up. In a similar study in Denmark, no decreased risk of dying was found. Both of these studies did not actually measure or monitor vitamin C levels in blood or diet. But the third and fourth studies I discovered did. In the EPIC-Norfolk study of over 19,000 men and women (aged 45 - 79), higher plasma levels of vitamin C significantly lowered mortality risk over a period of 4 years. A similar test of over 16,000 people also found that the as serum levels of vitamin C went up, risk of mortality went down.

I take these studies with a grain of... vitamin C. Yes, something is definitely going on here. And I'm sure vitamin C is responsible for some of the effect. It could also be that people who take vitamin supplements are performing an affirmation of their intention to be healthy and that they back it up with several other life-extending habits, like better overall nutrition and exercise.

102.

And then there is my Aunt Grace, who at this writing is 97, still rooting for the Yankees, and, to the best of my knowledge, has never swallowed a vitamin pill in her life.

Thanks for reading my book!

If you liked it, please let others know by reviewing it on Amazon, Goodreads, your own website...or just by telling your friends! Reviews mean an awful lot to a writer. Your support will help keep books like this coming. Thank you!

And if you came across things you didn't like, or things you expected to see but didn't, please let me know. You can write me through the contact portal at my website, **DominickBosco. com.**

Don't miss the next book in this series!

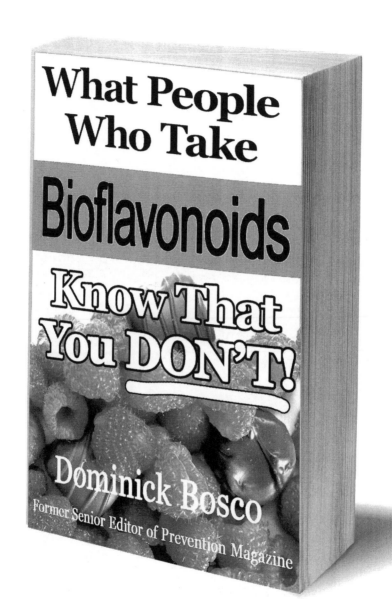

What People Who Take

Bioflavonoids

Know That You DON'T!

Dominick Bosco

Former Senior Editor of Prevention Magazine

Coming Soon!

Don't miss the next book in this series!

If you'd like to get insider info about my next books, the best way is to check out my website:

DominickBosco.com

I'll be offering free previews, advance notice on sales and giveaways, and new info on supplements.

Don't miss out!

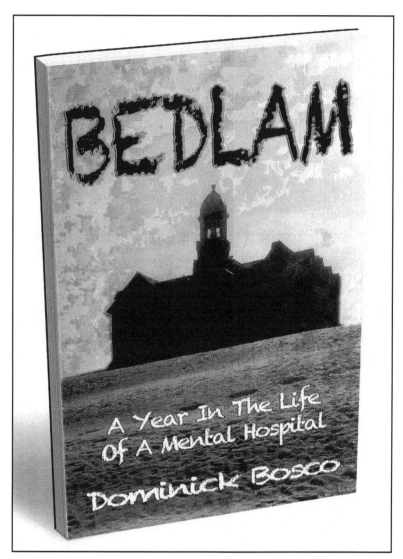

BEDLAM

A Year In The Life Of A Mental Hospital

by Dominick Bosco

"Educational, uplifting, heartbreaking. What more could you want from a delicious read?"

--S'Parks' 5-star Amazon review

"An eye-opening experience. A troubling book, difficult to put down...."

--Library Journal

"By the time I reached the final chapter I found myself wishing there was more. I didn't want the story to have ended."

-- from the foreword by Katherine Broderick Anderson

Available NOW on Amazon

in print or for Kindle

Made in the USA
Middletown, DE
27 December 2015